Psoas Release Party

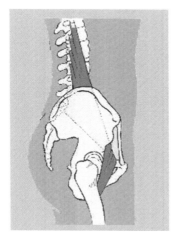

Learn To Understand The Feeling And Healing Of Your Pain!

By Jonathan FitzGordon

Other books in this series:
Sciatica/Piriformis Syndrome
The Spine: An Introduction To The Central Channel
The Exercises of CoreWalking

Cover Illustation: Frank Morris

TABLE OF CONTENTS

FOUR VIEWS OF THE PSOAS MUSCLE

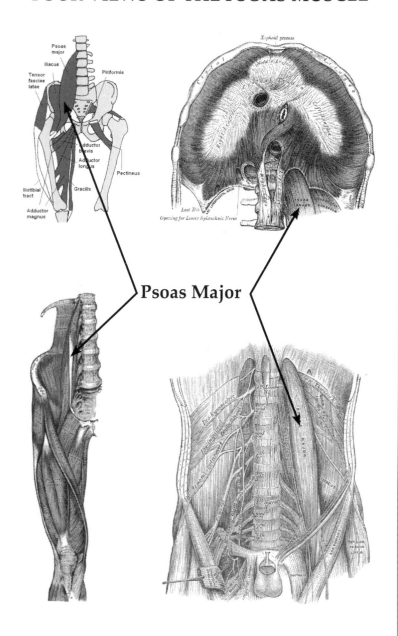

Psoas Major

I. THE WONDER MUSCLE

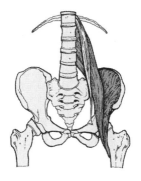

As a yoga teacher, I was taught to stretch people, but it wasn't long before I began to come across people who didn't seem to be served by stretching. They would come to class with dogged regularity, but their hips or hamstrings or whatever they hoped to lengthen never seemed to acquiesce. I came to realize that a muscle that is full of tension cannot be stretched free of that tension. In certain cases we must learn to release the tension and/or trauma from a muscle in order to get to the point where we can stretch it.

Deep in the bowl of the pelvis lies the psoas major, the body's most important muscle, which many people have never heard of. This muscle, my favorite, is both the main engine of movement and the main recipient/warehouse for trauma.

The human body is a miraculous creation, an intricately designed machine in which every part plays a specific role in trying to keep the body in a state of balance. It is a balance that crosses many spectrums—muscular, skeletal, emotional, physiological, etc.—and this elusive balance requires a great deal of harmony among disparate parts of the body.

THE PSOAS MAJOR

At the center of it all is the iliopsoas muscle group, three muscles lining the core of the body on either side. The psoas major is the body's main hip flexor and one of only two muscles connecting the lower and upper body. When healthy, the psoas major in front and the piriformis across the back help us stand upright in a perfect state of balance. The psoas attaches along the lower spine and comes down to cross over the rim of the pelvis before it moves backward again to insert on the back half of the inner thigh. The tension that the psoas creates across the rim of the pelvis as it moves backward at its top and bottom is critical to healthy upright posture.

The second muscle of the iliopsoas is the iliacus, which has a similar job to the psoas. The iliacus muscle lines the bowl of the pelvis and meets the psoas major to form a common tendon that inserts on the back half of the inner thigh.

The third muscle of the iliopsoas muscle group is a very interesting muscle called the psoas minor. It is considered to be a devolving muscle—according to anatomy books, only 50 percent of the population has this muscle.

The psoas major connects at six points—it attaches at the base of the rib cage and the top of the lower back. It connects to the outer edge of the first four vertebrae of the lumbar spine, which is the lower back, and to the front of these vertebrae as well as the front of the 12th thoracic vertebra, which is at the base of the rib cage, and it crosses over the front of the pelvis and goes backward to attach on the back half of the inner thigh, on a bony projection called the lesser trochanter. As a result the psoas spans and affects many joints.

There are many important joints or junctures in the body, but I always return to four particular ones that involve the psoas. These are the two femoral joints, where each leg meets the hip bones of the pelvis; the lumbosacral, where the pelvis meets the spine; and the thoracolumbar, where the lower (lumbar) and middle back

Thoracolumbar

Lumbosacral

(thoracic) meet. This last spot is where I see the most fundamental postural collapse in most of my clients. Improper alignment of the skeletal system always leads to imbalances in the muscular system, and vice versa.

The placement of the pelvis determines a great deal of what happens in the legs, trunk and arms. Again, the psoas is one of only two muscles that connect the upper and lower body, and even though it doesn't 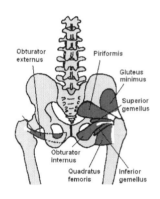 connect to the pelvis (57 other muscles do), it exerts a profound influence over its alignment. The other muscle is the piriformis, which attaches the leg to the sacrum. The psoas connects the body across the front and the piriformis at the back. These two muscles, when working well, perform a balancing act that allows for successful upright posture. A problem with one of these muscles always involves a problem with the other as well.

When the psoas is in an unhappy state, there are a host of physical conditions that can be connected to its issues—lower-back pain, hip pain, groin pain, bladder problems, constipation, poor circulation, leg-length discrepancy, scoliosis, bad menstrual cramps, and the list goes on and on. For instance, a chronically tight psoas on both sides pulls the vertebrae of the lower back forward, which can lead to pain due to compression of the joints and discs of the lower spine. If the psoas is tight on just one side, it can trigger a contraction of that entire side, causing one leg to be shorter than the other; it may even lead to the curvature of the spine known as scoliosis. This book will give you a clear understanding of how and why the psoas is involved with all of these issues.

THE PSOAS AND BREATHING

In addition to bridging the legs and the trunk, your psoas is intimately connected to breathing, as the diaphragm muscle, the main muscle of respiration, has ligaments that wrap around the top of the psoas and two long attachments, called crura, that come down to insert on the first three

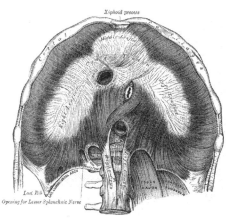

vertebrae of the lower spine. This means that every breath resonates in some way with the psoas, and the movement or lack of movement in the psoas influences each breath.

THE PSOAS AND FLEXION

The psoas is the body's main hip flexor, which is why it is the main muscle of walking, but it plays a deeper—and maybe more important role—within the nervous system. Flexors are muscles that bring one body part closer to another. The act of flexing has a relationship to the body's nervous system through our fear response. Our sympathetic nervous system, which is responsible for our flight-or-fight response, manifests through flexion; like all animals in the wild, when startled or afraid, we automatically react. The psoas is involved in any of these reactions.

Life is traumatic, and this is not necessarily a bad thing. From the big trauma of being born and taking our first breath to the lesser traumas of day-to-day life, we are here to be traumatized, and to varying degrees, we develop an inner support system to heal. Like the pulsing of the heart and the ebb and flow of the tides, the body's trauma/healing interplay is as natural as breathing.

What concerns me is when the nervous system

doesn't successfully integrate a traumatic event, very often manifesting this through pain and injury to the psoas. When this happens, the trauma can become trapped in the body. This imbalance can register in many ways—emotional, postural, energetic—but it will always involve the psoas, and from my perspective, the road to relief from trauma must go through the psoas.

HOW DOES IT WORK?

The body is divisible into many systems, only some of which I will touch on here. My main concern is movement, and all movement in the body involves the skeletal system, the muscular system and the nervous system. Your bones hold you up, and your muscles move you; your nerves tell your muscles to move your bones. What we want to do is align the bones to free the nerve pathways so that they can tell the muscles to move the bones in the most efficient way. As we will see, the psoas major is intimately involved in all three of these systems.

Balance begins in the core of the body. Over the past few years, "the core" has become an abused phrase, but it deserves its due. A great deal of my interest in body mechanics stems from the difficulty of our evolution from quadrupedal to bipedal beings. This shift has not been smooth.

A four-legged animal doesn't require the same balancing act from its skeleton that we do and as a result doesn't require the same core stability. It is much easier to balance a four-legged table than a two-legged table. Our ability to stand upright puts untold stresses on our muscles, bones and joints, and it is the tone and balance of the core that can and will allow for ease in the standing body.

Finding this balance requires a specific alignment of muscles and bones. For the bones to align, our muscles must have a certain amount of tone to keep everything in place.

WHY DOES IT GO WRONG?

Our posture is determined and affected by many things. In the first place, we learn by imitation, so we truly are who we come from. As we will see, the way in which we make our way to walking has a great deal of influence on our later movement pattern. Accidents, injuries and the way we heal from them often have a lasting effect on the body, as do so many other factors.

Most important is the idea that the body is a specifically designed machine in which every piece plays a part. It has been my experience that people simply don't know how they operate. Most clients that come to me are experts in something and could probably talk at length about their field. But very few can tell me exactly where or how their head is supposed to sit on top of their body. Most of us do not know that our overall health has a great deal to do with how our head sits atop our spine. The way our head sits influences our posture. And proper posture is interchangeable with proper movement and health.

Understanding the body's mechanics is a key component of our ability to institute change. If you knew that your psoas was meant to align in a specific way, and you were able to tell that alignment felt right and seemed to take stress off your legs or back, you might be willing to do it. That is why a general understanding of anatomy is a key part of my approach to helping people make the necessary changes in the body.

Different reasons factor into an individual need for either stretching or releasing muscles. Hopefully, over the course of reading this book you will understand the need for both. The exercise section is geared toward releasing the psoas, but there are a few delicious stretches thrown in for when the psoas is ready to get long and strong.

And finally, your psoas is the tenderloin or filet mignon. In a quadruped, the psoas isn't really called on to work that much, as it doesn't actually touch the pelvis. Its function as a support structure really comes into play when tension is brought to it as we stand up and the psoas is pulled taut over the rim of the pelvis.

The distinction between quadrupedal and bipedal animals is very interesting. The movement from being four-legged creatures to two-legged ones has not been particularly successful. And it is something that we must deal with in an effort to prevent our bodies from breaking down as we get through our 80 to 100 years.

Homo sapien is the name of our genus. This translates as "the one who knows he knows." I love that translation because I think it is our knowing that gives us so much trouble. An animal in the wild does not suffer trauma in the same way that we do. It is our conscious thinking that allows the trauma to live in the body the way it does.

Homo sapien is only 200,000 years old. We are very young and just starting to figure these things out. I'd like to think that if we're around for another 100,000 years, we might just get this psoas and standing thing right.

II. THE PSOAS IN INFANCY

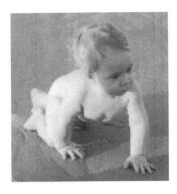

Allow me a word or two about babies. It is so easy to see the little blobs that lie before us as just that. Cute little blobs to be cooed at and passed around for others to see. But they are so much more than that. The newborn brain is developing at a rapid pace, and physical development in the first year profoundly affects us for the rest of our life. There are many specific physical markers all babies are meant to hit along the road to standing and walking.

The journey that we all take to become a standing individual imprints many patterns that might never go away. These patterns take hold through repetition, and if we don't think at some point of changing them, there is no reason why they won't be ours forever. If you buy into that idea, we should take some time and look at the process of early development and the awakening of the psoas, which is not called upon to work until you begin to sit up and stand. In a baby's first six months, the psoas lies dormant because the legs do not bear weight, and it is actually important that they don't at this time.

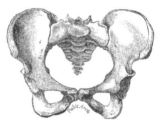

NINE IN, NINE OUT

There is a school of thought that says we are born premature—about nine months too soon—but we have to come out because the head and brain are growing too big for the human pelvis. In the process of being born, there is a big head that has to get through a little pelvis. While your bones are pretty soft as a baby, the bones of the cranium are separate, and they overlap with each other when you're born. If you touch the head of a week-old baby, you can usually feel the ridges of the cranium before they separate into a flat head.

The adult pelvis is made up of four bones: the two hip bones, the sacrum, and the coccyx, or tail bone. In utero, the pelvis contains anywhere from

12 to 14 bones. The hip bones in utero, and for about anywhere from nine months to a year after birth, are each made up of three separate bones (the ilium, the ischium and the pubis). Over the course of the first year, these

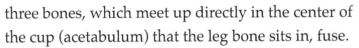

three bones, which meet up directly in the center of the cup (acetabulum) that the leg bone sits in, fuse.

But if these three bones haven't fused into one bone yet and you put weight on the foot and then take that weight up into that hip bone, you're not doing it a service. The hip is not designed to bear weight until those bones fuse into one solid structure. I bring this up to elucidate a very important aspect of baby handling. Babies should never be stood up on their legs until they are ready to stand by themselves.

The neighborhood where we have our yoga studio is baby central. Walk into a restaurant and it is a given that you will see parents with children, very often young babies, being stood up on their feet and held aloft by their hands. I'm not one to proselytize in restaurants, but the friends to whom I have discreetly mentioned this always say how much it seems that their babies love this feeling. It is hard to argue with the look of glee that is on their faces. It must be an amazing feeling to be standing on your parents' thighs and be at Mommy and Daddy's eye level.

Imagine, though, if you didn't stand your child up until he or she could stand on their own. After about a year (give or take) of sitting, crawling and exploring, a child will pull himself up to stand for the first time on a solid hip and confident footing.

This is all a key part of natural psoas development. Allowing the body to develop naturally is a key ingredient of coordination and grace in adulthood. Newborns should really spend as much time on their belly as possible when not being held, and babies should be allowed to find their movement markers on their own. The act of sitting up is one of life's first and most important achievements. How great would it be if children could find their way there on their own?

There is an emotional component to this process. Let's say a baby who has never been sat up finally— at around six months—sits on its own. It knows how it got there and in turn knows how to move back to square one. The inverse is that the sat-up baby has little control over its fate.

Now, these are pet peeves of mine, but they are connected to the intrinsic development of the psoas. As mentioned earlier, the psoas lies dormant in infancy and awakens in the baby's first movement from hands and knees to sitting. For many babies, sitting up and beginning to crawl often coincide. And crawling is the next key phase in psoas development. With crawling comes the lengthening and toning that prepare the muscles to help the bones bear weight as the young skeleton makes its first forays into the world of standing. There is a similar emotional connection for babies on their bellies as opposed to babies on their backs. A baby on its belly is a grounded object—it might not be able to crawl yet, but it can touch finger and toes to the floor and have a grounded sense of a protected umbilicus. Babies on their backs are kind of lost in space, unable to do anything but flail their hands and feet to no avail.

Babies should be left on the belly as much as possible. If you sit a baby up, it doesn't really know how it got there, and it doesn't really know how to get back onto either its back or belly. But if the baby sits up on its own at the very first moment that it can, it understands how it got there, and more importantly, it knows how to get back to where it was, so it's in a very safe and grounded place.

These movements, from on the floor to sitting to crawling to standing, reflect the awakening of the psoas. Crawling before standing is particularly key, as that really develops tone and length of the psoas.

Ideally, the progression is belly to sitting up to crawling to creeping, which is walking around by holding onto furniture, and then to standing. These things can't take too long. In fact, the longer it takes, the better. The more time spent at each given stage, the more the psoas will be toned and the more prepared the bones will be to bear weight for baby's first steps.

Sitting up, standing, creeping, and finally walking create a true awakening of the psoas as a support structure, and, in many ways, it will never relax again.

III. THE PSOAS IS A PULLEY

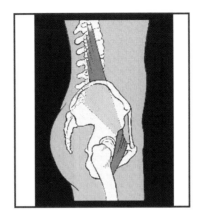

Everything changed for the psoas when we began to walk on two feet. The psoas is the filet mignon, or tenderloin, because in a quadruped it doesn't touch the pelvis during its journey from thigh to spine. When we stood up to walk on two feet, everything shifted. The big butt muscle, gluteus maximus, along with the hamstrings pulled down on the back of the pelvis to draw the spine upright. When the spine sits on top of the pelvis the psoas crosses the front rim of the pubis at the front.

As the trunk is pulled up on top of a level pelvis, the psoas tones because it attaches on the back of the inner thigh bone. The tension created in the psoas as the spine becomes vertical draws the vertebrae of the lower spine forward, effectively creating the oh-so-important lumbar curve. This small curve in the lower back, born in the ascent to bipedalism, is the weight-bearing element that allows us to stand upright and balance the rib cage and head on top of the pelvis and legs. The lumbar curve is what allows us to stand for prolonged periods of time and is one of the essential differences between humans and our nearest primate ancestors.

Once we get to standing, there are numerous opposing forces working to hold us up. We have only two muscles that connect the leg to the spine: the psoas and the piriformis. They both attach on the thigh bone. The psoas attaches on the back of the inside of the thigh, and then it travels forward and up across the pubis. The piriformis attaches on back of the outside of the thigh and then moves slightly up to attach on the inside of the sacrum. These two muscles basically strap the spine to the leg at the front and back of the body. The piriformis muscle is often involved with pain related to the sciatic nerve (the subject of my next e-book).

Energetically, the body splits at the pelvis, with the legs rooting down to the earth and the spine lengthening to the sky. As mentioned, the gluteus maximus and hamstrings pulled down so that the spine could stand up. The psoas, which lived horizontally when we walked on all fours, is now vertical—and crucial to the spine's ability to find extension.

Also, the psoas and another group of muscles, the erector spinea muscles, interact to help the spine lengthen up. One of the things I love about anatomy is you can learn so much from looking at the names of things. The erector spinea muscles are, like the name promises, the erectors of the spine. They connect behind the psoas and run all the way up to the cranium, lengthening the spine and creating critical support for the head. These muscles work in a chain, and they all need to be able to work together for effective use.

When the psoas engages to pull the lumbar vertebrae forward, the erector spinea respond by lengthening up the back. When one or both of the psoas become tight, pulling the lower back forward into too much of a curve, the erector muscles shorten and lose tone. When these lower erectors lose tone, the upper erectors lose tone as well. This can create compression in the bones of the lower spine and can also lead to kyphosis, a common rounding of the upper back (sometimes referred to as a dowager's hump). Ideally, when the inner thigh pulls back and the tension is brought across the front rim of the pelvis, the downward pull of the front of the spine will allow an upward pull of the erectors, a counterbalancing action that provides support up through the head and the neck.

In general, a key to a healthy body is finding the balance between flexion and extension. The back muscles of the body are extensors (gluteus maximus, erector spinea); they provide extension that helps us to stand and lengthen up. The front muscles of the body (including the psoas) are flexors; they provide contraction that enables us to walk, run and survive (flexors connect to our fight-or-flight response in the nervous system). As we will soon see, most of us have this balance backward, living with posture that has basically reversed the body's natural order.

Figuring out how to successfully employ all of these muscles will allow for the body to begin to work as it was designed. The body is a machine, a series of arches, hinges and pulleys, and the psoas fits into the mechanical model as a pulley. When the psoas contracts, pulling across the front rim of the pelvis, the hip bone can act as the pulley, multiplying the natural force generated by the psoas. When the tight, weak or misaligned psoas fails to create this tension, lower-back pain may arise as the lumbar vertebrae are pulled forward and become compressed in the back.

If I had a 500-pound weight sitting on the floor,

I wouldn't be able to pick it up with my hands. But if I attach a pulley to the ceiling, run a rope from the weight to the pulley, I will then, in all likelihood, be able to take the weight up off the floor without a great deal of difficulty. The psoas is the rope, and the hip bone is the pulley. But the psoas has to be properly aligned for the pulley system to work, and in that respect the psoas must live in the back plane of the body.

The power of the psoas is based on its placement. Unfortunately, it can't place itself properly on its own. In fact, certain muscles (which we will look at in the next chapter) must be toned for the psoas to be perfectly positioned.

Ideally, we can stand with good posture, as seen in the diagram on the left. This means the legs are aligned under the hips, and the head and shoulders are stacked above the hips. Then your psoas can act as a pulley.

In doing so, the psoas provides for the reciprocal upward lift of the erector spinea muscles that lengthen the spine up the back.

However, for many of us, the thighs sink forward, pulling the pelvis down at the back.

Does the diagram on the right look familiar? You can see that the lower back shortens as the upper back falls backward to compensate. Welcome to 98 percent of the people who come to me for help. In this position, the psoas is drawn slightly forward and open at its base, thus losing any tension that a pulley system might provide.

Remember that the back of the body contains the extensors and the front body has the flexors. Well, when we look at the two pictures above, you can see that the guy on the left embodies this balance, while the guy on the right has actually turned his flexors into extensors and his extensors into flexors.

Come up to stand and take note of your posture and get a feeling for the way you normally stand. Odds are the muscles of your thighs and butt are working way more than they need to. Stand with your feet parallel and try to shift your thighs backwards releasing your butt and untucking the pelvis slightly. Try and imagine how this action moves the psoas into the back plane of the body. Turn the feet out and tuck the pelvis under again and see where the insertion of the psoas goes. It moves to the front plane of the body. When this happens, there is no longer any tension created by the pull of psoas over the rim of the pelvis, and the support offered by the pulley action disappears.

Play with this and see if you can feel the difference in the support of the spine with the butt tucked under and the feet splayed out against the reverse of sticking the butt out and turning the feet in. Feel free to exaggerate in both directions to get a feeling for what you are doing. It is great to do this in front of a mirror and watch for the effect on the body. With the butt tucked under and the thighs sinking forward, the lower back collapses, as does the neck, forcing the head slightly forward. Stick your butt out and see the difference as the lower back and neck both lengthen in a good way, bringing support to the spine.

Every time you find the proper placement of the pelvis, you are feeling the power of the psoas. And that feeling is the pulley action as the inner thigh pulls down and the psoas draws the lumbar spine forward allowing the spinal muscle to lengthen the spine to vertical.

From my perspective, this most common misalignment—thighs leaning forward, pulling the psoas into the front plane of the body— is responsible for a great deal of our shoulder, head and neck soreness. Fortunately, developing the action of the psoas as a pulley is a relatively easy way to help ourselves find proper standing alignment.

IV. MUSCLES THAT SUPPORT THE PSOAS

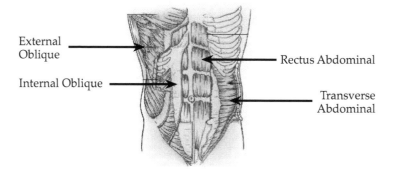

External Oblique

Internal Oblique

Rectus Abdominal

Transverse Abdominal

THE HOLY TRINITY

Our bones hold us up, and our muscles move us. I am always trying to simplify and reduce things to easily understood sound bites. But it is often more complicated. In this section, we are going to look at three muscle groups, the holy trinity, that work to support the ideal positioning of the psoas. For the psoas to be the wonder muscle that it is designed to be, it must be properly situated at its top and bottom, and it can't find that placement by itself.

These groups are the adductors, muscles of the inner thigh; the levator ani, muscles of the pelvic floor; and the eight abdominal muscles.

THE INNER THIGHS

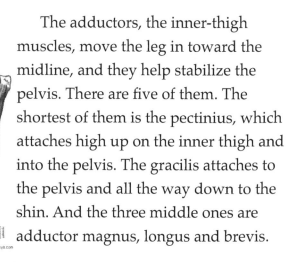

The adductors, the inner-thigh muscles, move the leg in toward the midline, and they help stabilize the pelvis. There are five of them. The shortest of them is the pectinius, which attaches high up on the inner thigh and into the pelvis. The gracilis attaches to the pelvis and all the way down to the shin. And the three middle ones are adductor magnus, longus and brevis.

All of these muscles attach around the pubic bone. But the adductor magnus, the biggest of them, has one head that attaches to one of your sit bones, the ischeal tuboroscity. Interestingly, that makes this muscle responsible for not just moving your leg to the midline but also assists with internal rotation. And that ability to rotate the leg in is an absolute key to stabilizing and setting the psoas.

Proper tone of the adductors allows for the psoas to live in the back plane of the body, which, as we've seen already, is vital to good posture.

MUSCLE BALANCE

Let's take a moment to look at the concept of muscle balance. Every group of muscles has an opposite that it works with to provide stability, support and efficient movement. The opposite of the inner thighs are the outer thighs, the abductors. In all areas of the body, these muscle pairs are meant to be balanced, working in concert with all the other muscles around them to provide equal or reciprocal energy for proper use.

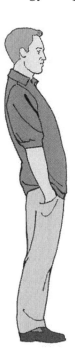

There are classic imbalances resulting from poor posture due to the unsuccessful employment of the psoas. In the neck, one of the most common misalignments—the ears living forward of the shoulders—creates a strong imbalance between muscles on the front and back of the neck. Most people tend to be closed in the front of their upper chest, so those muscles are short and tight and the back muscles are long and weak. It starts at the base of the body—if the shinbones and calves settle backward, the thighs are forced forward, drawing the pelvis down and causing the lower back to shorten (no pulley). As a result, the upper back falls backward and the upper chest rounds in, taking the head and neck with it.

We are supposed to be evenly balanced, with

the upper chest as equally wide and broad as the upper back. Our inner and outer thighs have their own reasons why they are rarely a happy couple. One of them returns us to early childhood. Just as sitting up and crawling awaken the psoas, these movements also are a significant vehicle for inner-thigh development.

Crawling employs a dynamic stretching of the psoas and optimal use of the young adductor muscles. If employed over a length of time, when a baby pulls him- or herself up to stand, there will be beautiful balance and tone between the inner and outer thigh. To this end, it is not in a baby's interest to walk early. In fact, barring neurological problems, the longer a baby crawls the better, allowing time for the growth of core coordination. But crawling is only one issue.

POSTURAL IMBALANCE

Very few of us are aligned to allow for balance between the inner and outer thighs. If you tend to stand and walk with your feet turned out, which I'd say is a large part of the population, your inner thigh would by necessity be weaker than the outer thigh—due to the position of the foot and pelvis, the inner leg turns out and is no longer in a position to work effectively.

Many of us stand this way because our parents stood this way, and so much of our learning is by imitation. Unfortunately, generation after generation of bad posture will haunt us until we get it right. Think about your parents and siblings and try to figure out whose posture and body type you inherited, if one more than the other. Figure out who you move and walk like and then try to decipher why that might be the case. It might not be a parent. It could be an older sibling that you bonded with or an aunt whom you loved dearly. That which we become is a tapestry of so many threads.

So what does this imbalance bring us? Outer-thigh dominance tends to pull us toward external rotation, which really complicates things. Your deep gluteal muscles are designed to function as both internal and external rotators. The problem is that these designs are based on the ideal. Should you stand up straight and have both feet pointing forward and not too far apart, the gluteals would be positioned in such a way that they could serve both functions. Half of their span would be toward the front plane of the body, and half would be toward the back.

Try standing with the feet together, the eyes closed, and the big buttock muscle, gluteus maximus, relaxed, and see if you can sense what is going on deep inside. The gluteals are dynamically going back and forth in search of a stable place between inner and outer rotation. Now turn the feet out and move them apart. It is likely that the pelvis shuts down energetically, its joints become somewhat locked, and the inner rotation of the thighs, which is always key to the psoas, is gone.

Building proper tone in the inner thighs is imperative if we want to get our legs under our pelvis for proper posture. The psoas can't live in the back plane of the body without the help of balanced leg muscles.

THE PELVIC FLOOR

The muscles of the pelvic floor are called the levator ani. Three muscles form a sling at the bottom of the pelvis that connects the tailbone to the pubis. This mass of muscle, about the thickness of your palm, is responsible for holding the pelvis organs in place and for control of rectal and urogenital function. Not only are these muscles bearing a lot of weight from above; they are also pierced by orifices that weaken the pelvic floor merely by their presence. Continence is high on my list of priorities, and the pelvic floor and continence are dancing partners that we must train and respect. Because these muscles are involved with your eliminative functioning, they have more resting tone than any other muscle in the body and are almost always active—or you'd be peeing all night long.

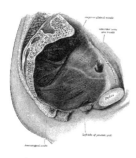

The pelvis and the muscles surrounding it serve a role unique to bipedal mammals. Just like the psoas, which is relatively dormant in quadrupeds (hence the tenderness of its loin) but wakes up when standing upright brings it into positive tension across the rim of the pelvis, the pelvic floor has a greatly different role in the biped. If you think of a dog or a cat or a horse, their pelvis is the back wall of the body rather than the floor. This leaves the organs in a dog to rest on the belly. In standing bipeds, the organs sit right on top of this muscle group, which frankly has enough to do without its newfound responsibility. Kegels exercises were created to help women with post-pregnancy incontinence issues. I think these exercises are the most important exercises any of us can do (we will learn to build the inner thighs and do kegels in the third e-book in this series).

When you have strength in the pelvic floor, what you're getting is a stable pelvis, and the stability of the pelvis allows for the psoas to move across the rim of the pelvis and have a proper, strong, toned gliding action on its journey to being a pulley.

Muscles of the Trunk

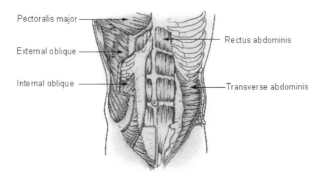

The last group of muscles we'll look at is the abdominals, equally important for many different reasons. You have eight abdominal muscles—four pairs. All four sets of these muscles move in different directions.

As we look at a cross section of the trunk (below), notice the way the abdominal muscles are

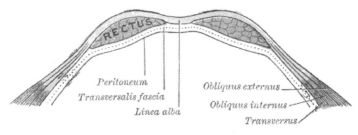

all connected, both through the tendons and the fascia.

The deepest of them is the transverse abdominus. It wraps from the back to the front, meeting at the linea alba. We often refer to the transverse as one muscle, but it is two muscles that meet in the middle. This deep muscle when properly toned, provides a great deal of support to the lumbar spine.

The next layer of abdominal muscles consists of the internal and external obliques, which are angled in opposite directions. These muscles help in twisting, rotating, bending and flexing the trunk and are also active when we exhale.

THE SIX-PACK

The third set of abs is the rectus abdominus, the "six-pack." This pair of muscles runs vertically, connecting at the pubis at its base and the sternum and three ribs at its top. An anatomical aside about the six-pack: The body has interesting and different ways of compensating for dilemmas of length and space. The length between the pelvis and the rib cage is really too big for one long muscle to provide support. As a result we have tendinous insertions that fall between what are actually ten small muscles. So we really build ten-packs, but we only see six of them. This pack is formed when we make these individual muscles big enough so that they essentially pop out from the tendons that surround them. Muscle is designed to stretch; tendons are not.

HARD MUSCLE IS BAD

I have a clear image in my head of the guy on TV selling his six-minute abs program. He looks out at the camera with his six-pack jutting proud, but his shoulders are hunched over toward his pelvis as though he couldn't stand up straight if he wanted to. I always wonder if he is bent over to make his muscles pop or if that is his natural and proud posture.

I guess this might look good to some, but I'd like to take a moment to explain the nature of what happens to your muscles as you build them. Blood flows into muscles, passing through the endless number of fibers that make up an individual muscle. The way we build muscle is by creating micro tears in the muscle fibers; as they heal or repair, the body overcompensates in a way, replacing the damaged tissue and adding more, for protection against further damage. As we continue to build a muscle, the fibers need to have somewhere to go, and they begin laying down on top of one another. As more mass develops, the layering becomes denser and harder. At a certain density, blood flow will begin to become inhibited.

Just as the tight psoas results in back and other problems, a tight rectus can bring its own set of problems. Depending on the individual, breathing, digestion, circulation, and even the flow of nervous energy can be impaired.

The cultural arena of our body is a fascinating one. We have so many compensatory patterns due to the way we feel and look. We tuck our pelvis because we think our butt is too big, we hunch our shoulders to hide our breasts or because we don't like being tall. There are many more to add to this list, but I am really fascinated by the desire for six-pack abs. Our society lives in worship of the sit-up or crunch, thinking it is an express train to beauty.

Whether you think they are beautiful or not doesn't matter compared to knowing what they do and how they are connected to all of the other abdominal muscles. When we look at the cross section again it should become clear that because these muscles are connected to one another, they need to have equal tone. Imagine if one set were way stronger than the other, as tends to be the case with the rectus abdominus: As one muscle gets stronger, the other groups become weaker. We have to step back to find a new approach to balanced muscle building.

The fact that every muscle is designed to carry out a specific function has little bearing on what that muscle actually does. The brain might have a wish list in terms of a nervous response to a given stimulus, but a dominant muscle will take over ten out of ten times. With regard to the abs, it is the rectus abdominus that tends to engage at the expense of all the other abdominals.

These abs aid in breathing and help all movements of the trunk and pelvis, and for the purpose of the psoas they go a long way toward stabilizing the vertebrae and reducing stress on the spine.

Hopefully you are beginning to see that if these muscles are connected, they need to have equal tone. If they don't, and one of the four groups is stronger than the other, the other three groups are going to get weaker. The other, more pleasant scenario is that it is almost guaranteed that your psoas can find its proper place if these three muscle groups, the holy trinity of the inner thighs, pelvic floor and the abdominals, are toned and living in their proper places.

V. THE EFFECTS OF A TIGHT PSOAS

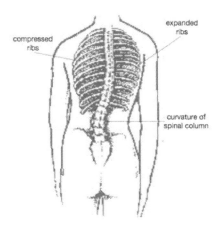

A happy psoas major is a long muscle that lives deep in the bowl of the pelvis, creating a shelf of sorts for the abdominal contents on both sides of the body.

Let's begin our journey into dysfunction by tightening the psoas on the right side. Everyone is tighter on one side of the body—stronger and tighter on one side and looser and weaker on the other; they both have their advantages and disadvantages.

Let's see what happens when the right psoas tightens. The right leg is pulled up into the right hip, restricting movement. The psoas has a bit of external rotation when it is flexed, and this shows in the tight hip by turning out the right foot. Another possibility is that the tight psoas both pulls the right

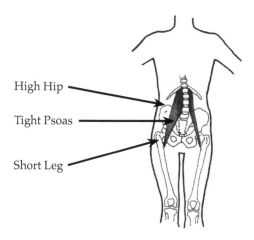

High Hip

Tight Psoas

Short Leg

hip up and draws the bottom rib down.

Have you ever noticed that one of your legs is shorter than the other? Almost everybody is going to fall into this category. But maybe one in a million people actually has the bones of one leg shorter than the other. Most often it is the tightness of the psoas muscle that creates this discrepancy in leg length.

It is easy to go through life and never even realize that one of your legs is shorter than the other, and some people find out about it in odd ways, like going to a tailor and when their pants come back hemmed they see that one leg is shorter than the other.

How well do you know your posture? Does one of your legs turn out more than the other? If it does, that as well is likely the pull of a tight psoas.

Beyond leg-length discrepancy there is an endless array of dysfunctional possibilities for the psoas. Imagine if both psoas are tight. What will happen in this case is the femurs get jammed up into the hip socket, and the psoas pulls the lumbar vertebrae too far forward, creating an excessive curve. And that excessive lumbar curve finds compensation in what's called a kyphosis, where the upper back pulls in opposition to the lower back. I see this pattern in 75 percent of my clients to one degree or another.

A tight psoas on one side means that the leg on that side will be pulled tight into the hip socket. This is one of the hallmarks of what we in yoga call tight hips. The psoas isn't the only contributor to tight hips, but it is almost always involved. Any time there is this kind of environment in the hips, movement is going to be restricted, and the leg and pelvis will tend to move as a unit rather than moving independently as designed. Functional movement in our body is dependent on freely moving joints. And the movement in our joints is reciprocal with other joints in the body. There are specific correlations between the hips and the ankles and the knees and the lower back. If the movement at the hip is restricted, as it will be with a tight psoas, that movement is going to have to come from some other joints, and this is one of the reasons why we have such a high incidence of knee and lumbar injuries. Movement that should occur in the pelvis and hips comes either from above or below and negatively affects those joints.

Many people believe that scoliosis is due to shortness or tightness in the psoas. Let's take a look at how that might work. You have the psoas on two sides, but imagine if only one is tight. If I pull down on this psoas, it's very easy to see how the pelvis might twist and torque forward. As a result of the pelvis twisting and torquing, the rest of the spine is going to have to twist along with it—there's really no way to avoid that.

Besides the spine moving, another result will be that muscles begin to move in opposition; even ribs can get involved. In a really bad case of scoliosis you might see that the upper ribs are so affected that you get what appears to be a hunchback as the ribs are pulled back.

Compensation is possibly the most important part of understanding and unraveling what it is we're trying to do in the body. If my car breaks down, that's it—it doesn't go anywhere. If I get a flat tire, I'm stuck with my flat until I get my flat fixed. But if my body breaks down, it is designed to compensate.

The muscle that compensates, unfortunately, has to take on a lesser role in its original function and often can't work as well because it is doing two jobs rather than one. If I hurt the inside of my foot, the muscles of the inside of my foot do not work as well, and the muscles of the outside of my foot have to help. That, by nature, is going to diminish the quality of the muscles of the outside of the foot.

That is going on everywhere, but it's not such a bad thing if we heal and then reverse the course of compensation. But we are rarely that conscious, and very often these compensatory patterns become part of the body and stay as part of the body.

If you start to learn about your body and how it works, you come to understand the power of the psoas and realize how opening, stretching and releasing it can bring amazing health to the body; then there's a real incentive to find this health.

VI. THE PSOAS AND THE ORGANS

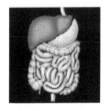

The psoas exerts a great influence on the contents of the trunk. When you have a long and toned psoas, it lives down in the bowl of the pelvis, and it creates a container for the organs with the pelvic floor below, the rectus abdominus in front and the diaphragm above providing support and protection for everything within.

The contents of the trunk, your organs, should live in or above the bowl of the pelvis. A short, tight psoas gets in the way of this possibility. The tightness of the psoas pulls the lumbar vertebrae and the psoas forward. If the abdominal muscles lack tone, the trunk's contents are pushed forward; if there is too much tone, they can get squished in between the psoas and the strong abs.

Have you ever seen a pregnant woman who is so big that she looks like she's going to have twins yet she is carrying an average-sized baby? The fetus and the abdominal contents can be pushed forward due to psoas tightness, and it might appear that she is going to have a giant baby.

Have you ever seen a skinny person who has a potbelly, but they don't have a lot of fat on their body? Again, the tightness of the psoas can push the abdominal contents forward, resulting in the appearance of a potbelly.

WALKING IS FALLING

We often come back to the psoas as the main muscle of walking. When we are functioning correctly, the entire body is toned and stimulated by proper walking pattern. When you learn how to walk properly, the body's natural healing processes can kick into gear.

Walking is a core event initiated by the nervous system in response to falling. Let's say the right leg is in front as you are moving forward through space. The brain tells the psoas of the back or left leg to initiate movement to catch you before you fall. Walking is, at its core, falling endlessly forward through life trying to find yourself in the effortless wave of gravity's flow.

Instead of that ideal, most of us tend to walk or fall backward, leading with the legs, placing the feet down ahead of you, instead of falling forward through the feet. This pattern fails to take advantage of the psoas during walking.

Walking from the psoas initiates a spinal twist with each step that is facilitated by the alternating movement of the arms and the legs. When the right leg and hip go forward the right arm releases backward. At the same time, the left leg and hip go backward and the left arm goes forward. This results in a spinal twist with every step that allows for and encourages the proper movement in the pelvis and spinal joints, twists and cleanses the internal organs, and affords better access to the breath through a more effective interplay of the psoas and diaphragm. One of the key benefits of the FitzGordon Method core walking program is wellness through movement. Good gait is preventative medicine.

When your psoas begins to walk you through life, it is drawn down and back through the inner thigh. Your lumbar spine is pulled forward. When you switch legs, the opposite happens. Add the arms to that, because the arms and the legs move in symmetrical opposition, and you get a powerful rotation through the lumbar spine that is stimulated and initiated by the psoas.

This affects everything in the area. Very specifically, it stimulates and massages the intestines and the bladder and really begins to show you the connection of the psoas to digestive and eliminative health.

The psoas lives right next door to the bladder. Many people wake up to urinate a lot of times over the course of a night. Very often, it is a short, tight psoas pressing against the bladder that creates the environment for that to happen, and hopefully releasing can help you out of that.

A short and tight psoas can also restrict the flow of blood and create circulation problems. The abdominal aorta, which supplies blood to the pelvis abdomen and legs, splits into the left and right iliac arteries which follow the path of the psoas down towards the leg. Poor circulation in the feet and toes can be a common indicator of psoas problems.

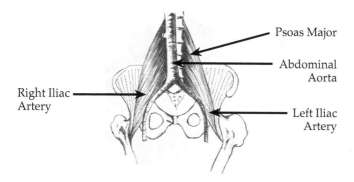

Let's look at the psoas's connection to breath and the diaphragm, which can have a profound effect on the nervous system. Fascia, ligaments and tendons all connect the diaphragm and the psoas.

There are two tendons, called crura, that come down from the diaphragm to attach on the lumbar spine alongside the psoas attachments; the ligament of the diaphragm wraps around the top of the psoas, where it connects into the 12th thoracic vertebra These connections mean that the psoas is involved with every breath and the diaphragm is involved with every step.

The pelvic floor and the diaphragm are synergistic. What that means is that they work together. Every time you inhale, and this is in a healthy, ideal body, the pelvic floor and the diaphragm both lower fractionally. And they both rise with every exhale.

Connect this to the breath and the synergistic working of the diaphragm and the pelvic floor, and you start to get a really amazing bit of movement in the body. With every inhale the psoas draws back into the bowl of the pelvis as the rectus abdominus draws forward, and the diaphragm and pelvic floor lower. With every exhale everything retracts, the diaphragm and the pelvic floor move up, and the psoas and the rectus draw back in.

This gives us a window into the work of the psoas as a hydraulic pump in concert with the synchronized pumping of the diaphragm and the pelvic floor. This stimulates and massages all the organs and all the bones and moves fluids through the entire trunk.

VII. THE PSOAS AND THE NERVOUS SYSTEM

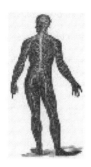

The nervous system is the body's information gatherer, storage center, and control system. It collects info, analyzes it and initiates the proper response. The central nervous system, which is the big kahuna, includes the brain and spinal chord. The peripheral nervous system connects the central nervous system to the body via nerves that come out of the central nervous system.

There are a number of divisions within the nervous system. Your peripheral nervous system has a motor division, and within that motor division, there are two other divisions, the somatic and the autonomic systems. Within the autonomic systems come two subsystems that we will focus on.

These are the sympathetic nervous system and the parasympathetic nervous system. The sympathetic is the system of excitation, and the parasympathetic is the system of relaxation. Both systems innervate the same organs and act in opposition to maintain homeostasis, the Greek word for staying stable or staying the same. For example, when you are scared, the sympathetic system causes your heart to beat faster; when the fear has passed, the parasympathetic system reverses this effect. Homeostasis, the search for balance between excitation and relaxation, is at the heart of our well-being.

We move now from the purely mechanical workings of the psoas and dive into its deeper role in the body.

We know that nerves tell muscles to move bones. But there is also an emotional side as well; the nervous system is constantly working to maintain harmony in the realm of fear, worry and safety. The fear response plays a large role in our movement and postural capabilities. The main action of this response is flexion, so we return always to the psoas, the body's main hip flexor. Any time we are involved with the sympathetic nervous system, the psoas will be involved, which is fine as long as the journey into fear is balanced by an alternate response from the parasympathetic system.

Life is fear, and our relationship to fear is a large part of what determines the nature of our health, our posture, our muscle tone, even our emotional tone—maybe especially our emotional tone. And fear is flexion. We flex for security; we flex because we need to in reaction to the fears that come up in life. It doesn't matter what these actions of safety or protection are—running, fighting, hiding—they're all flexion.

And we always come back to the psoas. All of these acts of flexion are great if they're balanced by a happy interaction with the parasympathetic nervous system. They're designed to work together.

Let me give you an example of the interaction of these two systems. Let's say it's the middle of August and you walk outside onto the street and it's 100 degrees. The first thing that happens is your internal body temperature begins to rise. As that happens, your nervous system takes note, and the sympathetic nervous system kicks into action to produce sweat to cool down the body and reduce internal temperature.

As soon as the body temperature is lowered, the parasympathetic nervous system comes into play to reduce the sweat. This happy interplay is constantly going on in your body. Let's say you cooled down enough to stop sweating but then get on an air-conditioned bus. The same mini drama plays out in the nervous system, seeking balance of the internal environment.

What concerns us is when something creates an imbalance between these two systems. This imbalance can register emotionally, posturally, or energetically, but it will always involve the psoas, and from my perspective, the road to relief from trauma must go through the psoas.

Now I'll share a story of what it is like to get stuck in the sympathetic nervous system. Let's say you have a boss whom you hate, but you have to see him every day at work. You get in the car in the morning at 8:00 and settle in for the hour's drive to work. Life is good. You listen to the radio, maybe talk on the phone. You're feeling good.

As soon as you get to work, you pull into the parking lot and shut the ignition off, and all of a sudden you feel the engagement of the sympathetic nervous system. Maybe it's a little white light across your lower back; maybe it's a tingling up and down your spine; maybe your mouth goes dry. Whatever it is, you're no longer happy. You have just gone from ease to dis-ease.

But that's okay, because you and your boss work in different areas in the office. You pass by his office, you say hello, he grunts hello and you relax a little—the parasympathetic steps in, says, Oh, okay, we can bring balance back, let's chill out.

You have to do it again at lunch, and you have to do it again when you leave work, but that's all right, that's the natural process, the natural balance. But let's change the scenario a little bit and say that your boss does not have a separate office and you work at a desk next to him. What happens then? At 9:00 a.m., the car turns off, and the sympathetic nervous system turns on and does not release until you leave. You walk on eggshells, and everything that happens during the day creates a startle response. You're always waiting for that reaction. You're always waiting in fear, and as a result the sympathetic nervous system stays engaged and will never release.

This story can be applied to many different scenarios, most profoundly to war zones, car accidents, destructive home environments, muggings, etc. Any trauma can create this imbalance in the nervous system. The specific event or trauma doesn't matter. It is the body's ability to process the trauma that determines what comes next. Essentially it is the body's ability to discharge the trauma that allows for a healthy fear response and in turn a better chance to achieve homeostasis, which is where the psoas release comes in. The body, when traumatized, will process the trauma, but it can't always process it immediately and it can't always process it well.

To release the psoas is to allow for a letting-go of long-held trauma, whatever that trauma might be. If the stuff of our lives is still living in the body, we want to try to come up with a way of letting it go. And for me, releasing the psoas is the key first step on a long journey to a balanced body. It has been my experience that you can't stretch a muscle that is full of tension, whether that tension is postural or emotional. You must first learn to step back and release these muscles before you can dive into a beautiful journey of building length and tone in free and easy muscles.

CHAPTER VIII: RELEASES

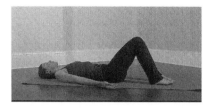

WHAT IS A RELEASE?

The exercises in this manual are as much about exploring your psoas and your pelvis—specifically your pelvis's relation to the legs as they meet the hip sockets and the sacrum where it meets the lumbar spine—as they are about healing. With the FitzGordon Method, healing cannot begin without awareness. Settle into these explorations to come to a better understanding of how your body works.

Physical, emotional and postural health are predicated on a body having supple joints. We are essentially drying up from the moment we are born, and a great deal of our struggle in aging is about staying lubricated. Tight, constricted joints inhibit lubrication. Again, if you are reading this you likely have some tight joints. Every one of these releases is intended to bring movement and clarity to the hip joint.

Finally, before you begin, know that releases are about not doing. Want less and you will get more.

Trauma is a strange bedfellow. It has no interest in hanging around. You just have to find the subtle means of letting it leave.

The following exercises can be done in sequence if you have the time but are also effective individually. For instance, someone who experiences hip pain while walking can stop on any street corner to do the Foot on a Block exercise that comes third in this series. Temporary relief can go a long way toward permanent relief when it comes to retraining the nervous system to believe that pain can be abated.

What you will need:

- A mat.

- A belt.

- A blanket.

- Three yoga blocks or equivalent-size books.

- A tennis ball.

- An orange or its equivalent.

CONSTRUCTIVE REST POSITION (CRP)

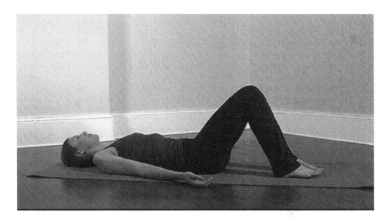

This is the main psoas release that we work with. It is a gravitational release of the psoas that allows the force of gravity to have its way with the contents of the trunk and the deep core.

- Lie on your back with your knees bent and your heels situated 12 to 16 inches away from your pelvis, in line with your sit bones.

- You can tie a belt around the middle of the thighs. This is a good thing to do, especially if you are weak in the inner thighs. You want to be able to really let go here and not have to think too much about the position of your legs.

- Then do nothing. You want to allow the body to let whatever happens to it come and go. Discomfort arises from conditioned muscular patterns. Try to allow the body to release rather than shift or move when unpleasant sensations arise.

- You are hoping to feel sensation that is something you can sit with and allow it to pass.

- Try to do this for 15 minutes a day, twice a day—in the morning and at night. If you have time, longer sessions are advisable.

But we are not here to suffer. If sensations come up and you feel that you just have to move, feel free to move, then come back to where you were and try again. It's possible that you'll do this exercise and not feel anything; that is fine also.

TENNIS BALL UNDER FOOT

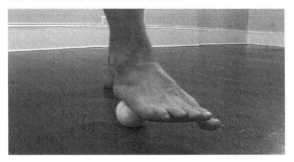

Technically, this is not a psoas release, but it is a gift to the body any way you look at it. This is great before or after constructive rest as well as anytime during the day. I recommend keeping a tennis ball in a shoe box under your desk; that will keep the ball from squirting away while you roll.

• Place a tennis ball under your right foot.

• Spend a minute or two rolling the ball under the foot. You can be gentle, or you can apply more pressure. The choice is yours.

Step off of the tennis ball and bend over your legs. You can check in with your body and see if you feel that the right leg seems a bit longer and looser. Feel free to scan the whole body in this fashion. There is a thick pad of connective tissue on the sole of the foot called the plantar fascia. By releasing the fascia on the underside of the right foot, you effectively release the entire right side of the body.

FOOT ON A BLOCK

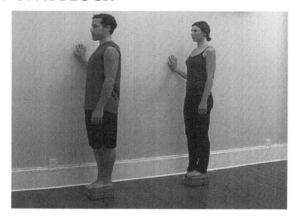

This is a gravitational release of the psoas. This exercise is not limited to your house. If you have hip or groin pain when walking, feel free to stop at every corner and dangle one foot off of the curb while holding on to a lamp post.

- Place a block eight to ten inches from a wall.

- Step the left foot up on the block, allowing the right foot to hang down between the block and the wall. Place your right arm on the wall to help you stabilize the upper body.

- Keep the hips level and rotate the inner thighs back and apart—stick out your butt a bit, and feel like you can let the leg go from the base of the rib cage, the top of the psoas.

- Once you are comfortable with the leg hanging out of the hip, you can move the leg half an inch forward and back as slowly and steadily as possible. Half an inch is a very short distance.

- Let the leg dangle this way for 30 seconds or until the standing hip has done enough.

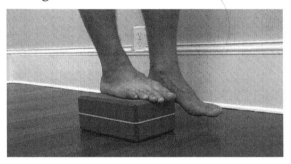

- Switch sides and tune in to which side is tighter. Do the second side for the same length of time that you did on the first side.

- Repeat for a second time on the tighter side.

DIFFERENTIATING LEG FROM TRUNK

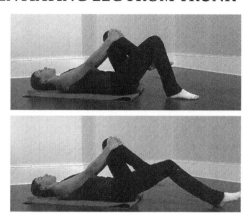

- Bend the left knee and interlace your fingers at the top of the shin. Hold the leg out at arm's length. Extend the other leg. Pay attention to the hip socket—only move your leg, not the pelvis.

- Bring tone to the pelvic floor and the low belly and do your best to stabilize the trunk.

- Extend the right leg out slowly. It doesn't have to extend completely.

- Slowly lift the right knee up, drawing the heel toward the hip and keeping the left heel on the floor with the foot flexed.

- Maintaining a stable trunk, extend the right leg out again.

- Repeat ten times on each side if possible. Feel free to start with as few as three times.

SUB OCCIPITALS

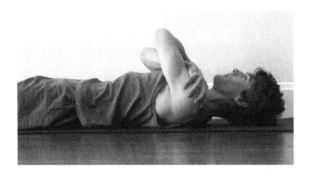

The sub occipital muscles connect the base of the skull to the top of the spine and are the only muscles in the body with an energetic connection to the eyes. They tend to be chronically short.

- Lie flat on your back and bring a small natural arch to your lower back. The legs should be straight; you can put a blanket under the knees if there is any strain on the lower back.

- Raise your arms to the sky, pulling your shoulder blades away from the floor. Try to let the upper spine settle onto the ground. Grasp each shoulder with the opposite hand.

- Lengthen the back of the neck as much as you can without closing off or creating discomfort at the front of the throat.

- Stay for three minutes to start, and try to build up to five minutes.

RELEASING ARMS

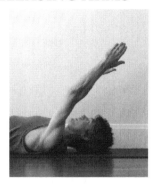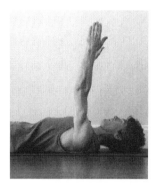

This exercise works on the ability to articulate the arms separately from the trunk.

- Lie flat on your back and bring your arms up, with the fingers pointing toward the ceiling.

- Begin to lower the arms over head, trying to keep the rib cage and spine from moving.

- Only go as far as you can go without the trunk moving. Be willing to start slowly and increase the range of motion over time.

- The eyes and head can follow the arms in movement.

CACTUS

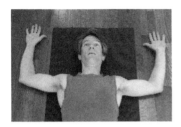 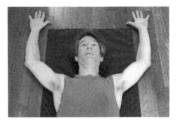

This falls somewhere between a release and a stretch and is not nearly as benign as some of these explorations. In fact, this can be very intense, though you won't be doing much.

- Lie flat on your back. If it is not comfortable to lie with the legs straight, roll up a blanket and place it under the knees. This will release the hamstrings and reduce the strain on the lower back.

- Bring your arms out to the side and bend your elbows to form a right angle with the arms.

- Lengthen the back of the neck and allow the spine to soften toward the floor. The lower back and neck should each have a gentle arch, but ideally the rest of the spine should have contact with the floor. Move very slowly.

- Once you get your spine into a good place, bring your awareness to the forearms, wrists and hands. Try to open the hands, extending the wrists and the fingers. Move very slowly.

- Once you get the arm to a good place return to the spine. Go back and forth between the two and allow the back of the body to lengthen, soften, and release.

BLOCK LUNGES

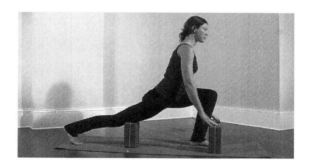

This is a release of both the quadriceps and the psoas. Sometimes the quadriceps muscles are so tight, there is no getting to the psoas until we release the quads a bit. You'll need three blocks for this.

- Positioned on your hands and knees or in Downward Facing Dog, step the right foot forward in between your hands. Two blocks will be for your hands by the front foot.

- Place the third block underneath the quadriceps muscle just above the knee, at the base of the thigh.

- Tuck the back toes and let the weight of the body fall onto the block. Do your best to keep the heel of the back foot pointing straight up toward the ceiling.

- The front leg and hip should not be under any strain. Feel free to make adjustments, turning the foot out or stepping the foot wider.

- You need to stay for 90 seconds to get the full benefits of this pose.

RELEASING HANDS AND KNEES

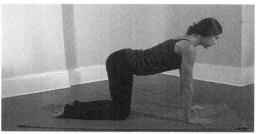

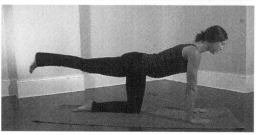

This exercise explores the ability of the leg to separate from the pelvis and the spine.

- Start on your hands and knees with the hips over the knees and the wrists underneath the shoulders.

- Bring gentle tone to the pelvic floor and the lower belly and try to extend your right leg back, bringing the leg level with the trunk.

- Keep your awareness on the lower back and the pelvis stabilizing the trunk to release the leg.

As always, these are experiential exercises where you try to get a feeling for what the body is doing. The tighter psoas will be the side that can't move without pulling the pelvis and the spine with it.

TONING

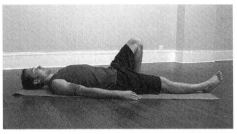

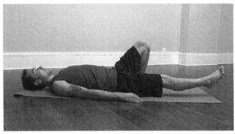

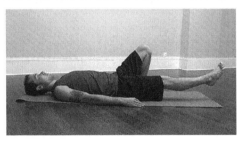

The following exercise works the psoas more than most of these explorations. Proceed slowly, and don't overdo it in the beginning.

- Begin in constructive rest. Extend the right leg straight out.

- Press the left foot down into the floor to help the right leg lift up two inches.

- Lift the right leg three or four inches higher,

and then lower it back to two inches off the floor.

- Repeat five times if possible, keeping the pelvis and spine stable. The only thing working is the leg.

- Switch sides.

Once you are comfortable taking the leg up and down, begin again by pressing the opposite foot into the floor. One variation is to move the leg from side to side, and another is to move the leg on a diagonal, staying within a three- or four-inch range of motion.

Note: Three inches is a very short distance.

TIGHT-HIP RELEASE

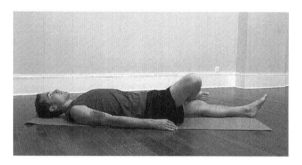

This is meant as a passive release for extremely tight hips. If your knee is higher than a 45-degree angle from the floor when you assume this position, this exercise is for you.

- Lie on your back with the legs straight out on the floor. Stabilize the trunk and bring the right foot as high up on the left thigh as possible.

- Allow the right knee to release toward the floor, keeping the trunk stable the entire time.

- Try to let the release come from both the inner and outer thigh as gravity takes the leg toward the floor.

- Stay for five minutes on each side if possible.

ORANGE THING

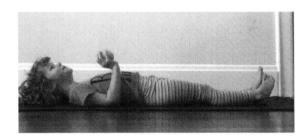

This is more for fun than anything else. Look at yourself in a mirror before and after you have done one side and see if notice a difference.

- Lay flat on your back with an orange or a ball of similar size sitting by your right hip.

- Roll the orange slowly back and forth from the heel of your palm to the fingertips.

- Pick up the orange and hold it in your open palm with the elbow on the floor and the palm facing the ceiling.

- Balance the orange on your palm for two or three minutes before stopping.

CHAPTER IX: STRETCHES

PSOAS STRETCH: LUNGE ON FLOOR

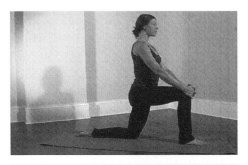

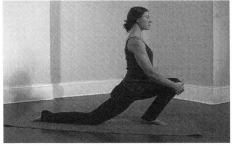

In this exercise we'll experience a dynamic stretch of the psoas.

• Start on your hands and knees and step the right foot forward in between your hands. Feel how all four corners of the trunk are pointing straight ahead. Try to maintain that alignment throughout the whole pose.*

• Interlace the fingers on the right knee. You can use the strength of the arms to help lengthen and extend the spine.

- We want the psoas to move back in space at the inner thigh and the lower back as the pelvis comes forward.

- Try to wrap the inner thigh of the right leg back, feeling the outer hip come forward. Take the low spine back and up, lengthening up all the way through the back of the neck, and allow the pelvis and the front knee to come forward if possible.

- Repeat on the second side.

*If the hips are tight, you're going to feel restricted as you come forward and try to work on squaring the hips toward the front. It's okay if the hips don't square completely. Don't worry about how deep the stretch is—you don't need to go deep. You just want to explore the basic idea of keeping the hips square and stretching your psoas.

PSOAS STRETCH: STANDING

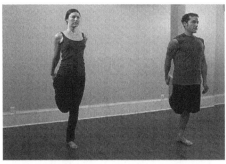

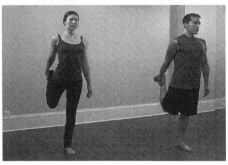

This is a classic standing stretch that also happens to be a deep stretch of the psoas—if it is done correctly. Feel free to use the wall to support yourself.

- Bend your right leg behind you and take hold of the right foot or ankle with your right hand. Bring your knees in line with one another, keeping the heel in line with your sit bone. If your outer hip is very tight it won't be easy to keep the knees in line.

- Pull the right leg behind you gently. Keep the pelvis and shoulders facing forward and upright the whole time.

- Keep the pelvic floor and the low belly strong as you try to pull the leg behind you through the balanced action of the inner and outer thigh.

If you have tight hips, it will be difficult to keep the legs aligned as you draw the right leg back. The knee will pull sideways, and it is imperative that you keep the legs in line. This is an issue with the iliotibial tract, or IT band, not the psoas, but as we know, everything is connected (no pun intended).

EXTENDED SIDE ANGLE

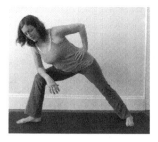 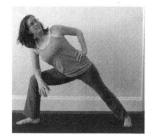

- Stand with the feet as far apart as is comfortable.

- Point the right foot and turn the left foot in a little.

- Bend the right knee, bringing the right forearm onto the right thigh and the left hand onto the left hip.

- Rotate your pelvis back, allowing the left

inner thigh to move back, lining up the outer left hip with the left ankle bone. This should pitch your upper body forward a little.

- Keeping the legs stable, try to extend the body trying to align the shoulder with the hip and ankle. This will require a lot of tone in the pelvic floor and lower abdomen. Don't allow the left thigh to move forward.

- Repeat on the second side.

TRIANGLE

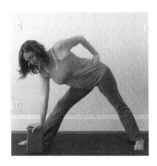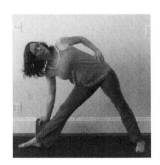

- Stand with the feet as far apart as is comfortable.

- Point the right foot and turn the left foot in 45 degrees.

- Place the right hand on a block on the outside of the right ankle, and bring the left hand to the hip.

- Rotate your pelvis back, allowing the left

inner thigh to move back in space, lining up the outer left hip with the left ankle bone. This should pitch your upper body forward a little. (picture on left)

- Keeping the left hip aligned with the left ankle, try to rotate the body and stack the shoulders on top of one another. You need open hips and a strong core to keep the thighs back and lift the trunk. Keep the belly strong and the spine steady as you go.

- Repeat on the second side.

DEEP LUNGE

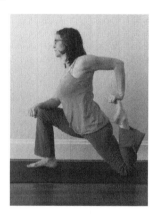

This is a very deep stretch of the psoas that shouldn't be attempted before the psoas feels long and strong and ready for more intense work.

- Starting on your hands and knees or in Downward Facing Dog, step the right foot forward.

- Place the right forearm on the right thigh.

- Bend the left leg and take hold of the left foot with the left hand.

- Draw the foot as close as possible to your left sit bone, trying to turn the pelvis and trunk to point forward.

- When you get your heel as close to the sit bone as possible, begin to move the hips forward. The right knee can go past the right ankle in the stretch.

- Try to keep the distance between the heel and the sit bone the same as you move the pelvis forward.

- Repeat on the second side.

WALL PLANK

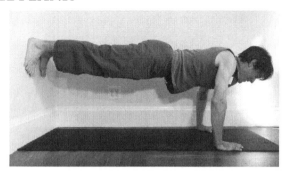

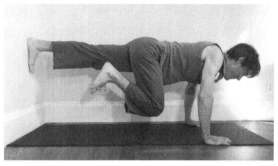

This is not easy.

- Lay prone on the floor with your feet up against the base of a wall. Bring your hands up alongside your chest.

- Straighten your arms, and walk your feet up the wall until they're level with your shoulders.

- If you are able to maintain this position, take the right foot off the wall and draw your right knee toward your chest. Maintain a stable trunk.

- Repeat with the left knee.

CHAPTER X: ACKNOWLEDGEMENTS

I have learned from so many people both in person and in print. Here is a short list of those who influenced this book:

Ida Rolf	Irene Dowd	Therese Bertherat
Liz Koch	John Friend	Bessel van der Kolk
Jenny Otto	Peter Levine	Sandra Jamrog
Tom Myers	Bonnie Bainbridge Cohen	

Many thanks to all of the students who have been patient with me on my path of learning; you have been my true teachers and my true guides.

Thanks as well to artists and models:

Chris Marx	Ida FitzGordon	Christopher Moore
Frank Morris	Jesse Kaminash	Mark Chamberlain
Heather Greer	Molly Fitzsimons	Caitlin FitzGordon

ART CREDITS

Illustrations:

Frank Morris - Cover, inside cover, pps 2, 8, 22, 26, 27, 31, 42

Grays Anatomy - pps 5, 10, 17, 18, 30, 35, 36

Mark Chamberlain - pp 49

Video Captures:

Heather Greer - pps 57, 59, 60, 62-64, 68, 70-72, 75, 77

Photographs:

Molly FitzSimons - pps 65-67, 73, 78-80, 82

www.CoreWalking.com

Made in the USA
Charleston, SC
06 April 2014